UNINFORMED CONSENT

UNINFORMED CONSENT

By Susan R. Urquhart

Thank you to Brian Lewis for helping to make this book a reality.

This is a work of non-fiction.

Publisher's Cataloging in Publication Data
Uninformed Consent / Susan R. Urquhart.

ISBN: 978-0-578-03492-8

First Edition

10 9 8 7 6 5 4 3 2 1

North Fork Publishing, LLC
Dexter, Michigan

Printed and bound in the United States.

For Brian,
I needed your love and support to spread my wings again.
You offered it mightily.

Contents

Preface

. . . .

They say everyone has a book in them. My someday book was going to be a children's story; I had planned to illustrate it, too. I had no intention that my book would be about hysterectomy; a subject about which I knew little.

But life presents its own path and my life took a negative turn with an elective surgery, strongly promoted by my former gynecologist of ten years, twelve years ago. Because I was a woman of a certain age, my former gynecologist also insisted on the removal of my ovaries, called a Bilateral Salpingo

Oophorectomy—more accurately a castration adjunct to the Total Abdominal Hysterectomy, to avoid the very slight risk of ovarian cancer. There is none in my family.

I was surprised with the results of the surgery; I went into a tailspin—spiraling downward to a place I had never been before; I plummeted into a state of severe depression. This was such an about face for me; my husband Brian was worried about me as well as my family and friends. I was worried, also; I didn't know who I was; I was scared.

My physician son and daughter-in-law and my good friend Toni got me in to see University of Michigan Reproductive Endocrinologist, Dr. John F. Randolph, Jr., who told me he would do what he could, but he could not completely replace my ovaries with drugs.

I learned that the damage done to my body was permanent and irrevocable. A sense of betrayal and rage consumed me. How could I have made these bad decisions?

I began writing; it was therapy. Over a ten year time frame, I shared my lessons learned, in missives; most of them were addressed to John Randolph. My goal is to educate; I am compelled to spare women from suffering my fate; this memoir is my attempt to do just that!

1 - The Antique Rocker

. . . .

The ratty, brown, antique wicker rocker in the sun room was never intended for two. It is my husband's favorite chair, in our favorite room, in our home.

They made the 1930's Haywood Wakefield chairs strong; they made them to last; the chair did hold two people, who rocked in it every night, for an entire year. The rocker was a refuge; with Brian's arms around me made it a safe place from all of my internal turmoil, where demons resided.

I would sit on his lap, with tears welling in my eyes and streaming down my face; afraid to be alone. The words that came out of my mouth were questions directed to Brian about my former physician's actions. Each night was the same; each night I repeated the same questions over and over to him. "She didn't understand, did she Brian?" "How could she have understood?" "Could she have known the cruelty of these procedures and still have done this to me?"

The sobbing, the questions, the loss of emotional and mental equilibrium, which permeated the core of my being, were not necessarily relegated to this nightly ritual. When I was able to sleep, I would always wake with the same fears and emotions instantly on my mind; if I couldn't sleep, they were with me all night; I arose sleepless at dawn; I carried them with me throughout the day until our rocking that evening.

I knew my emotional state teetered every minute on the edge of peril, I had no power to change. Every day and every night would be the same.

Our marriage was being tested as I never thought it would. He didn't have to tell me he grew tired of the topic of my surgery; or that he grew tired of my questions about my doctor's cruelty creeping into our every conversation. I also surmised he looked forward to the office as a respite from my emotional battle.

I had always been a woman who had made good decisions for herself and her family.

What caused me to make a bad decision on a surgery? A surgery I had resisted and avoided for ten years as a patient of my former gynecologist. There was a set of unfortunate circumstances; which I must admit, had to do in part with my strong, fiercely independent personality.

I thought I had chosen a reputable doctor. I asked good questions of her. I was unaware that her answers were fallacious. She had an unsullied reputation. I believed her untruths and deferred to her advice. I made the decision to proceed!

I thought it was my decision—my decision! I didn't even involve Brian in it! I didn't want to trouble anyone; I was a private person; to me this decision was something to be decided between my doctor and me, not anyone else; on hindsight, she coerced me, but because of our long term doctor-patient relationship, I had come to trust her, "in my best interest" was the phrase she repeatedly used. I decided I would get it behind me.

This is a story of trust, betrayal and greed; it is the story of a gynecologist who crossed over a line for personal gain.

It started in November of 1996, when I was 54 years old. According to my gynecologist my pelvic exam indicated that my fibroid tumor uterus had grown substantially since my exam a year earlier, to the size of a five month uterus, she said.

I received a phone call from her one month later in December. She said the ultrasound she ordered did not substantiate her claim. Did I still want to have the surgery? I gave her an emphatic "No". She insisted on an appointment in February, which she made herself that day.

I was annoyed! But my upbringing was to choose a good doctor and carefully follow instructions; I went to the appointment. It was a mistake that would send my life into a vortex of depression for 10 years.

I went to that February 7 appointment unaware; I came away having agreed to a surgery I had said "No" to many times before. I had agreed to the doctor's schedule of surgery in March, but my inner voice was worried! Was I moving too fast? Was this the right thing to do to my body? I was especially concerned about her wish to remove my ovaries; I knew they are a woman's gonads; I couldn't countenance removing them.

I did not follow my instincts—my woman's intuition! My lifelong practice of following a doctor's advice squelched that intuition. Brian and I have a friend, Les, who espouses a theory on life's near misses. I almost got away! If only I had listened to my inner woman.

One doesn't know the true measure of their mettle until it is put to the test; for both Brian and me the next chapter in our lives would be the measure of our mettle. Would it be our last chapter together? How would I come out of this myself? The strong, fierce independent person was gone. Would I ever come back? Would my life end as I knew it forever, or would I end it.

2-The Misdeed

. . . .

My surgeon came into my hospital room the morning after the surgery; she said everything went fine; my uterus weighed 680 gm, a near record for her! She said that it was good that I had gone ahead with the surgery. She then walked over to stand next to me; she bowed her head a little and said, "Your ovaries were normal."

What?! My heart sank.

I was sorry that I had gone along with her undue pressure for the removal of my normal ovaries—my mind raced back to the office visit where she had solicited my surgeries; I began to understand that undue pressure is an understatement.

At the February 7 office appointment I was sitting on the examining table naked except for a drape around me when she entered the room. She sat on the stool and said in a funny tone, "Now what are we going to do?" I said, "I don't know but I don't want to spend the rest of my life feeling the way I have lately."

Without asking how that was, and without reassuring me that it was only perimenopause, and self-limiting, she jumped up off the stool and began to circle the examining table! Each turn, she urged me to sign up for the surgery, which I had said "No" to, seven weeks before. She continued whirling around the table; every spin had a verbal spin on how great I was going to feel in just four weeks, if only she could sign me up that day.

I began to lose eye contact with her. My shoulders started to droop; my head went down at an angle. Finally she stopped in front of me for the first time and said, "Can I sign you up?" I could barely look at her but I muttered, "OK!"

We then talked about my perimenopausal ovaries as if they had no value. I told her that I knew that the ovaries continue to supply small amounts of the female hormones post menopause; I told her that the testosterone they continue to provide is essential for orgasm and a woman's sense of well being.

She nullified my legitimate arguments with the comment, "But I can put it all back." She promised me no less than three times that she could completely replace the function of my ovaries. I advised her that I didn't want to take the drugs as there was breast cancer in my family; I mentioned that I was at higher risk of breast cancer because my maternal grandmother died from it at age fifty.

She said, "The levels you take will be so low, it would never be a problem." I wondered how she could make that claim; I knew the jury was still out on that issue. But I fell silent—I didn't have enough information to refute her, but I wished that I did as I didn't want to replace my ovaries with drugs, I wanted to keep these important parts of my body.

When she lowered her head next to my hospital bed the morning after my surgery, I felt exploited. Now I saw an insincere woman; there was no remorse; in the flick of her eyelids, I glimpsed through her; I saw the real person; she had masterfully executed her plan—a hysterectomy with the oophorectomy; she understood the magnitude of what she had done to me; she did it with malice aforethought.

This rehearsed, staged scene, one no doubt that she had reenacted many times before, was a token, a nod to appease me, a gesture to ratify my loss. I found her performance troubling, callous and a sham. I was upset with myself; I was upset with her!

I hadn't come to terms with the removal of my organs. How could I? I had moved too fast with the surgery; the little inner voice bode correctly. Why had I not heeded it? I couldn't believe what I had allowed someone to do to me!

My part in the misdeed was part of my sorrow; but it was more than that causing my uneasiness. It was as if I was watching myself from a distance; it was—a disconnect, of body, soul and mind, more like another person lurking in my hospital room watching me and being me!

She discharged me from the hospital three days later—in the morning. I was given a pain killer and a dose of .0625 Premarin, which supposedly was to replace my removed ovaries. I told the her I wasn't sure that I wanted to take the Premarin, or even the pain killer; she insisted that I fill the prescriptions as she was sure I would need them.

Brian took me home and was donning his suit and tie; he planned to go to work! I felt sore and raw inside. I knew that I could not take care of myself. I started to scream at him. I shouted, "You have to stay home! You have to take care of me!" This was the beginning of my dependency!

3-The Visitor in My Body

. . . .

The physical pain abated in time only to be replaced by emotional pain and loss. I became despondent—detached! I lost all joy in the day; I had thoughts of suicide; I became sleep deprived; I was unable to read or concentrate, and crying was a daily affair.

It was three weeks after the surgery when I called my doctor for help the first time; not only was I emotionally bereft, I was experiencing vaginal soreness, bladder spasms and urinary incontinence. I spoke with a nurse, who talked to another doctor (my doctor was on vacation in Italy), who put me on the Estroderm patch, the same dose of estrogen, a different delivery system.

Three weeks later, at the six week check-up, I was again virtually naked on the examining table when my doctor entered the room. I glared at her; I said in an angry tone, "What happened to me?" She laughed at me; then she quipped in a mocking and patronizing tone, "Why, you're supposed to be feeling so much better! It's full bloom menopause, that's all. You'd be like this a year from now anyhow."

I emphatically retorted, "No! This isn't menopause!" I queried, "Why did you remove my ovaries?" She answered sarcastically, "You're mad at me, eh?" I answered, "I'm mad at myself and I'm mad at you, too!" She snapped, "You'll be all right. You'll get over it."

The way my doctor treated me at this appointment told me that I wasn't the first woman to complain to her. Her mockery and laughter were meant to disarm me; it was another performance, one which she plays out to the many women whom she has misused; as a way to dismiss them!

She prescribed a higher dose of estrogen; she prescribed testosterone for the first time. She told me it was OK to resume sex. I looked forward to sex with Brian; it had always been wonderful. But with my first attempt at intercourse I knew something was terribly wrong.

I went from a woman who would kick back and smile afterwards because the intimacy was so profound and satisfying, to a woman who now cried. I kept telling Brian, we have to do it over again!

Each try to regain what I had lost failed. I knew with certainty, in my heart of hearts, that something had been removed from my body which had been integral to my sexual pleasure—and it never again would be as profound an experience!

Seven weeks after my surgery Brian called my doctor. He told her my recovery was not what we had expected. He inquired if she removed my ovaries for her protection in the event that I later developed ovarian cancer. He said she volunteered, "I don't have to tell you, you're an attorney!"

Brian concluded her comment was an admission of guilt. I wondered how she knew he was an attorney as I don't remember ever mentioning that to her.

When my doctor pressured me for the surgery in early February, I asked if I would be well enough to participate in wedding of my son John, who was getting married at our home on May 17. She assured me that I could do anything in four weeks.

Eight weeks after the surgery, my loss of sleep was taking a dangerous turn; I was driving my 80 year old mother-in-law to a bridal shower, for my soon to be daughter-in-law, when I began having trouble driving. I had difficulty reading the road signs and reacting to them on time. I had always been so capable; I was the one everyone came to for help—never the one who needed it; and now I couldn't even drive my car.

I was always a feisty woman. I believed there was nothing I couldn't accomplish if I set my mind to it. When Brian and I bought a 240 acre farm in 1973, I was the one who took it over and turned it into a viable business—a Christmas tree farm.

I am not accustomed to disrespect from people, including doctors. So when I called my doctor's office the Monday morning after the shower, I insisted on speaking with my doctor. I angrily reproached her on the omissions and untruths in her preoperative counsel.

I said, "You should never have removed my ovaries!" She snapped at me, "You are the worst patient that I have ever had!" And she slammed the phone down and hung up on me. I was stunned.

I desperately needed help and now my doctor was through with me.

I was calling my doctor son Andrew who was in California every day now; I pleaded with him to help me. He told me that Lynda, my daughter-in-law, was better suited to help me, as this was her field. Lynda suggested I see Dr. John Randolph. With her and my friend Toni's help I was able to get in to see him in just two weeks.

I left a message for my doctor that I had an appointment with Dr. Randolph; she called me offering to get me in to see a Reproductive Endocrinologist at her hospital in as few as two weeks. I told her that Dr. Randolph came highly recommended and I was getting in to see him in as few as two weeks.

I was trying so hard to get the old me back, but I couldn't. It was like watching myself from the wings. I wondered if I would ever again be the strong woman I once was, the mother who raised two fine sons, the woman who ran our Christmas tree farm, the woman who was involved in the community, the woman who shares friendships with other women; the woman who was an equal partner with Brian.

The two weeks seemed like an eternity! Dr. Randolph was my hope. Brian obtained a copy of the December blood test and ultrasound from my former doctor which I would take to the appointment with Dr. Randolph.

Could he get the visitor, this intruder, this stranger, out of my body; could he bring the old me back? I was hoping that he had a potent elixir, a magic wand.

4-Maltreatment

. . . .

I was sitting fully clothed in a chair in the examining room when Dr. Randolph came into the room; he sat on a stool; I handed him the two pieces of white paper with the test results. He studied them; he shook his head from side to side and said, more to himself than to me, "But she is a good doctor!" I didn't understand the comment. He shared no more.

Dr. Randolph told me improvements in medical technology over the last ten years afforded the scientist a better view of the ovary; they learned the ovary doesn't lapse into quiescence at menopause; they learned that the ovary aids in circulation; it continues to supply a small amount of the female hormones. That is exactly what I had told my doctor! I was seething when Dr. Randolph told me that.

He explained he would do what he could, but he could not replace my ovaries entirely with drugs; this was the antithesis of what my doctor had told me. I knew ovaries don't cease to function. I gave this information to my doctor at the February appointment, when we talked about my ovaries, which she dismissed.

With each piece of information Dr. Randolph gave me, my anger built....

He told me the case had been poorly handled; he said that in six months or so I would look back on the trauma surrounding the surgery and laugh; I now knew there was a rough road ahead; I also knew there would never be laughter!

Dr. Randolph's candid, qualifying comments were sobering; my ovaries could not be replaced. I hoped, but now with cautioned optimism, that he could bring the old me back; it was a question I wrestled with, while choking back the burgeoning anger—what had I allowed someone to do to me?

I applied the double dose of the estrogen patches which he had prescribed; I readied myself for the wedding. Three days later, I slipped on the stunning mother of the groom's dress, which I had selected so carefully just before my surgery. It was now ill fitting, too large and hung unattractively on me.

I glimpsed at myself in the mirror to assess the damage. There was my red puffy face staring back at me; my brim filled, teary brown eyes looked like raccoon eyes with their dark circles; they had lost their sparkle. I had aged ten years in ten weeks! I reined in the tears, put some powder and a pasted a smile on my face and descended from my bedroom chamber to meet the guests.

My daughter-in-law, Deb, had done a wonderful job. We had a large white tent in the yard with little white lights all around that held our 250 guests; it even held a dance floor. It was enchanting! I made it through the wedding; I found a way to talk and enjoy the relatives and friends.

Monday morning I awoke with a rash over my entire body and immediately called Dr. Randolph's office. I was told to take a lesser dose of estrogen. I was to put on one patch every eighteen hours; I began to shake; I had heart palpitations, anxiety, and tremors when the estrogen levels fell. There was a long wait before I could put on the next patch which relieved these symptoms somewhat! It was the beginning of my long journey down.

I continued to suffer from vaginal soreness, urinary incontinence, urinary frequency, sleep deprivation, hot flashes, confusion, disorientation, depression and recent memory lapses. Lynda told me that I was suffering from hypoestrogenemia and hypoandrogenemia, which means my body had none of my ovarian estrogen and none of my ovarian androgens.

Two months after the surgery, I was beginning to put the pieces of the puzzle together.

On June 4, I sent a letter (I was so mixed up; Brian had to help me write the letter!) to my gynecologist, complaining of these consequences of which I had not been advised.

I wrote it to get some things off of my chest; I wrote it to help her become a better informed doctor.

I told her she needed to take more time in the future preparing a woman for her decision regarding prophylactic removal of her normal functioning ovaries—because ovaries are part of the balance of your endocrine system—and once they are gone they cannot be put back!

I wrote, "I am still wondering what I did to myself! I felt tremendous pressure from you to make that choice!" I suggested, "Either you are truly uninformed of the resultant trauma and suffering I experienced or you thought the risk of serious side effects so slight you decided not to discuss it with me."

The choice belongs to the patient; the role of the doctor is to make sure the patient's decision is an informed one. I told her that mine was not! I am ravaged. I went from a woman who couldn't get enough out of the day, to one who now snivels despondently in the corner.

I encouraged her to share my letter with other doctors for the benefit of future patients, who may then avoid the suffering I've had to endure.

It was an excellent letter, it came from my heart. I forwarded a blind copy to Dr. Randolph, with a cover letter.

In the cover letter, my first missive to John Randolph, I tell him I send it on to you as a teacher. Tell your students that women care greatly about their body parts; to remove them without valid reasons can be devastating to them; it can cause them to look back with anger.

I state, "The shock of this prophylactic surgery is uniform among women with functioning healthy ovaries. There is a sisterhood of us. I meet them in the pharmacy line. I'll be the spokesperson. I must comment to the teachers and policy makers."

Dr. Randolph was my lifeline. I was in almost daily contact with him at this point in time. Some of my conversations with Dr. Randolph were via his nurse, Carolyn—who was the go between. Dr. Randolph was incredibly kind to me; he gave me a lot of his time, but he had a practice to run. I think that is why I started to write to him—it removed the middle man—at least I knew he was getting my comments directly and unfiltered!

I was pleading with him to help me; he told me that I needed to stay on a drug for two weeks at a time, without other drugs in the mix, so we would have time to determine the most current drug's effectiveness.

This was time consuming; I had high hopes at the outset, with poor results at the end. We went through many different drugs; he started me on "Estraderm 0.1 mg patches times four with staggered replacement every three days." We then tried shots of Delestrogen 10 mg/ml, given @ 1 ML at his office; and then "Ogen 125 mg given by mouth twice a day to be titrated down from there as symptoms abate."

None of the drugs which he prescribed for me were doing anything to help. I was desperate.

I could not stop the tears. There was no gladness in my inner me. All of the things which had given me pleasure in life no longer made me happy. It was an effort to get out of bed in the morning—this kind of behavior—so out of character for a woman who had wished she had two lifetimes to live so that she could take in all of what life has to offer.

I was deflated. It was foreign to me. Before this surgery I could never have imagined depression. But I found myself caught in its tangled web; I didn't ever think I could care about things again. And I wondered if I even wanted to go on with my life. It had no meaning to me. I didn't care if I lived or died.

Intellectually I knew suicide wasn't the answer. But this wasn't an issue of just the mind... my emotions were raw—on the surface, exposed, and hurting.

No one in my direct bloodline had had a hysterectomy and an oophorectomy; I had no first hand experience with the surgeries. In my mother's day, when women had these surgeries, and had this reaction afterwards, it was inferred that there was something wrong with them; no one recognized the correlation of their bazaar behavior with the surgery, which was purported to be "good for them". They called it a nervous breakdown and they locked them up in a psychiatric ward! I was afraid it was a place where I was headed.

5-The Ruse Unravels

After my surgery, when I tried to resume my tree farm responsibilities, and I was inept, I could see people's bewilderment; a startled look came across their faces; like Ron's puzzled look the day I was about to leave his Duible Equipment, having signed the charge, but having left the much needed parts and my copy of the receipt on counter; or the look on Scott's face as I arrived at Bridgewater Tire, distraught and confused, having traveled miles in the wrong direction on the frequented route; they knew there was something different—something was wrong with me; only they weren't sure what it was.

When I took over managing our farm in the early 1980s, I was an anomaly—a woman at the helm of a male dominated business. Not only did some question my capability because of my gender, farming wasn't my background. And I was not playing the usual game; instead of cash crops I was planting trees.

My sons Andrew and John helped; and Brian helped, too, when he could! We planted Blue Spruce, Scotch Pine and Fraser Fir trees in the field at the corner of Steinbach and Jerusalem Roads outside of Ann Arbor.

We planted Kennebec potatoes in the wide rows between the small trees. We heard potatoes grown in sand were delicious. We used the tree planter to set the potatoes in the sandy field at that conspicuous corner. The traffic on the roads would slow down to watch what we were doing. The "real" farmers' laughter at the tree planting turned to hilarity with the arrival of the potato plants.

I expanded the fields of trees; I added irrigation where the varieties I planted required more water than we get in Michigan. The government subsidies on the farm enabled me to be paid for not planting corn, which helped finance the tree crop.

When the trees matured, we retrofitted our 100 year old gambrel roof barn, a former diary barn, into a Christmas Shop, where we sell our Christmas trees, gifts, ornaments, wreaths and garland. We give our customers a wagon ride through the rolling hills, over the streams and through the woods to their trees. On the way they may get a chance to meet my small flock of sheep and my llama, Willie.

The Interstate I 94 on/off ramp is three miles from our farm. The traffic on the roads adjacent to our farm is slowed now due to the crowds coming to get their trees. It's like Field of Dreams. So when I couldn't handle the daily responsibilities, we weren't sure what to do.

Roy, my main man, who has worked for me for twenty-five years, told me to go home and get better. There was nothing that I would have rather done--It took pluck, hard work—and more than a little luck; I bucked the odds; I succeeded where others might not have and now everything was in jeopardy.

I had always been so self sufficient. I never asked Brian to attend my doctor appointments before—I could handle anything—but I desperately needed him now. I asked Brian "Would you accompany me to the June 12, appointment with

Dr. Randolph?" I told him, "I feel like I am coming apart at the seams. I need you to go with me." He understood what had happened to me; I needed him to be there for me.

Brian confided to me, "You never needed me before! I am happy to support you when you need me." I didn't realize that my super self sufficiency left some holes in our relationship. I had left him out not realizing his support was good for both of us.

Dr. Randolph said that there was a loss of rugosity (folds in the vagina). He told me he wanted me off of everything now, except the Premarin Vaginal Cream. I was filled with trepidation. I didn't know if I could go without estrogen.

Brian and I had a fly fishing trip planned in late June. I was to call the office from the trip and let them know how I was doing. I called Dr. Randolph's office. I spoke to a nurse, but not Carolyn. I told her it hurt to have intercourse. I begged her to ask Dr. Randolph for permission to put on a patch. She told me that I could only take the Premarin Cream.

How could she be so cruel? My vagina felt like it was on fire—full of needles jostling about in every direction! I blurted out, "I am so uncomfortable! I don't think I can take this anymore!" She answered sharply, "Your Estrodial level is 1509! You had better start feeling better pretty soon!" I begged her, "Please, I don't think I can make it without putting on a patch." We hung up with no suitable resolution. I was going to have to be tough, and I was just beginning to realize how much so.

That night, Brian came in after fishing with his guide, and found me reading on his side of the bed, or what had been his side of the bed for 33 years. I was reading, but there was absolutely no retention. Brian told me to move over to my side. I told him, "I am on my side." He could not convince me otherwise. I would not move!

As he crawled between the covers on my side of the bed, he groused, "This is your side of the bed!" I responded in level voice, "I'm not on your side of the bed!" With that I switched off the reading light on his side of the bed!

I was sure I was right; he was in error... in the darkness, just to get in the last word he barked, "You're wrong, I'm on your side." To really get in the last word, I snarled loudly, "You're Wrong! Wrong!"

The next day I woke up on the wrong side of the bed.

We drove to Traverse City. Brian had won an expensive hand made Bamboo fly rod in a raffle; in fact he had won two rods a couple of years apart. It was like my brother Peter, who won a fully trained Labrador Retriever puppy; everyone but his wife knew he had purchased all of the raffle tickets.

We went to see Bob Summers, who builds these rods. He had a small, crowded and cluttered workshop behind his home. When I walked in, I was overwhelmed; my heart was pounding; I was shaking; I could barely breathe. I stepped outside! I wanted to go home.

Back home, I tried acupuncture. I was frightened to try it, but I was willing to chance it for the hope of some relief. It didn't help! Dr. Neu, an alternative medicine doctor and acupuncturist, told me that there was nothing he could do for me. He asked, "Why did you let your doctor remove your organs?" I sadly responded, "It is the biggest mistake of my entire lifetime!" He acknowledged as much.

I called Dr. Randolph. I pleaded for help. I was put back on the Estroderm patch just in time for another trip we had planned to San Francisco to attend the wedding of a son of friends. I couldn't keep it together. One night I couldn't join the festivities. Brian stayed with me; he held me in his arms, and on his lap, while I cried.

Again we went home and I had a deepening sense of desperation and hopelessness.

When I hadn't received a response from the letter which I sent to my doctor on June 4, I picked up a copy of my medical records on July 23. I showed them to Lynda. She flipped immediately to the pathology report where we discovered: "This is a 483 gm. 11 x 7 x 7.5 cm uterus with attached tubes and ovaries." Lynda said it was the equivalent of a twelve to fourteen week uterus, not a twenty week uterus which my doctor diagnosed.

We also discovered that my doctor's office had scheduled my surgery as a TAH-BSO (Total Abdominal Hysterectomy-Bilateral Salpingo Oophorectomy) on February 12, 1997, two weeks to the day prior to the appointment where my doctor said we would talk more about my ovaries—and where she coerced me into signing the consent form.

As the magnitude of my doctor's betrayal sunk in, I wanted my pound of flesh and was going to do anything to get it. I wrote to the State of Michigan Department of Consumer & Industry Services, Office of Health Services, Complaint and Allegation Division, on September 25, 1997, — I filed a formal complaint against my former gynecologist.

I wanted justice.

I beseeched Brian to find an attorney for me. I was adamant that I have legal representation! It was the only way to assuage me.

6-The Quest for Justice and Obstruction of Justice

. . . .

Brian was working on finding an attorney for me. He thought it would be good to have a woman represent me. He contacted two highly regarded female medical malpractice attorneys; neither of them would take the case; I had signed the consent form. One of them told Brian it was a "She said – she said case; that doctors lie; and jurors believe doctors."

Brian then found a male malpractice attorney who reviewed all the records. He met with us the week after Christmas in 1997. He told us, "The malpractice occurred on February 7, 1997. The act of malpractice was your doctor coercing you into agreeing to a surgery you had emphatically said 'No' to in a phone conversation seven weeks before."

He added, "She wanted another crack at you! She knew that she couldn't do it on the phone!" He told us he was willing to take the case. He said, "The case will have to be tried." He was convinced I would be a good witness; we should think about it as it would be a lot to go through, and if I was having problems emotionally, this could make it worse.

The following weekend Brian and I went to Chicago with friends. We stayed at our favorite small boutique hotel, the Raphael. On our shopping excursion, I was trying to memorize the street signs as we passed them so I could make the return trip to the Raphael by myself.

I couldn't do it. This was ten months after my surgery. I was afraid to leave Brian's side. This was another confirmation of why I had to do this—I was such a strong woman before; I owned and operated a tree farm, I was involved in the community, people wanted to be around me, now I couldn't even go out on my own. I called the attorney Monday morning. I told him I wanted to proceed.

Even if I had been told more of what I was going to experience with these surgeries, I would never have been able to comprehend the suffering. I was driven to get this woman in the courtroom. Now every waking minute of my postoperative life, I thought of nothing else!

If the damage hadn't been so permanent and irreversible; if she hadn't laughed at me—mocked me after I confronted her with my injuries; if she had admitted to a mistake; if she had then offered me her sincerest and deepest apology, it may been enough to palliate me, but she didn't do any of those things. I would get justice.

I had been seeing Dr. Randolph every four weeks since our first appointment on May 14, 1997. At our November 26, 1997, appointment he told me I looked better. He told me to make an appointment to see him in six months. Six months? Why so long? I was still floundering. I was adrift. I had never felt so alone and frightened in my entire lifetime. I had never needed anyone before, but here I was—completely inept and dependent. Could I make it with less of his help and involvement? I continued writing to him. I had to.

The first letter I wrote to Dr. Randolph since the June 5, 1997 cover letter, which accompanied a copy of my June 4, 1997 letter to my former doctor, was March 22, 1998. I told him:

I have many days where I cry and feel so down. I went into this surgery very much on top of my game mentally, physically and sexually. I lost my quickness, my humor, my vagina just stings on occasion, I leak urine as I go about the chores I enjoy, and my sexual response went from easily aroused and easily orgasmic—to neither post surgery.

In a May 4, 1998, letter, I told Dr. Randolph, I was better than I was the previous summer but my mental and physical state are light years from my pre surgery standard and I wonder if this is what I can expect with the BSO surgery, as drugs are no substitute for an ovary.

He mentioned at one of our meetings the previous fall that the most important sex organ is the brain. I told him you need more than a brain to have good sex; hormones and organs play a role as well.

I may have estrogen in my body but it is as if it is not connected—not being used—more like a faucet running at a certain volume—not like a complex metabolic organ supplying what is needed, in the correct amount and at the right time! And my testosterone is missing.

That was a horrible year for me. I was so angry and understandably so. The outcome of this elective surgery had catastrophic consequences for me and it appears its alleged necessity is indefensible.

I received a letter from the State dated May 8, 1998, regarding my complaint letter of September 25, 1997 against my surgeon, which stated, "The Michigan Health Professional Boards only have the authority to take disciplinary action against licensees for practicing below acceptable standards or for other violations that are enumerated in the Michigan Public Health Code."

They didn't acknowledge the reason for the surgery was bogus! All they cared about was whether the surgery met the Standard of Care; it is within the Standard of Care to unnecessarily castrate a woman!

My physician son tells me the Standard of Care is threshold medicine—it is the lowest standard of medicine that a physician may practice and still retain a license!

I was shocked and disillusioned! I had sent the State a copy of my medical records. The evidence was there in black and white. At a minimum it was clearly a misdiagnosis. I couldn't believe my lack of success at trying to right this wrong. I was thwarted at every turn in the road I pursued, but I wasn't going to give up.

Michigan Law requires that a plaintiff have an expert witness sign an Affidavit of Merit in order to commence a medical malpractice case. There is a two year statue of limitations from the date of the act of malpractice. There is a $250,000 cap on damages for pain and suffering, double that if a person's reproductive organs are removed, which mine were.

My attorney was looking for a "star" expert witness. He contacted several high profile expert witness physicians whom he thought might bring status to our case.

He found two with excellent reputations; they looked at my records; they both were disturbed that this surgery was performed, but neither was willing to sign the affidavit. After our expending several thousand dollars on potential witnesses, no one was willing to be the expert.

By signing the consent form I had made this a difficult case—it was the sticky wicket—that and the affidavit of merit! I have since learned that doctors who agree to testify against their colleagues, in any but the most egregious of cases, become ostracized by their peers; it is almost impossible to find a Michigan doctor willing to testify against another Michigan doctor.

It is within the Standard of Care to perform a TAH-BSO, albeit the lowest standard! Dr. Randolph told me it is within the Standard of Care to perform prophylactic oophorectomy adjunct to hysterectomy because the Specialty can not come to a consensus to change it. I suspect because the surgeries are lucrative, and doctors write the standards!

The attorney told me he didn't think we would be able to find an expert witness. He said it would be an expensive suit, with a small chance of remuneration! I was resolute; I wanted justice. I begged him to continue! I was not going to be dismissed so easily! I was committed; I must continue on this course. The anger inside of me wouldn't let me desist.

It was July of 1998 and the clock was running on the statute of limitations. It was a year and five months since the date of malpractice. Would there be no justice for me?

The pathology report had confirmed that my doctor made a misdiagnosis. Were my female organs of such little value that they could be removed for no reason without liability for monetary damages? Why wasn't there a doctor who would testify for me?

Would the same be true if a man's testicles were removed unnecessarily? It is as if women's sex organs have no value!

7-Lack of Due Process

. . . .

On February 7, 1999, the two year statute of limitations expired on my intended lawsuit. A few days before my attorney called to say that we could extend the statute by filing a six month extension, called a "notice of intent to sue", but we had better be ready as we could be called upon at any time to file it.

He recommended that I get on with my life. He thought the case futile—a waste of our money and his time! I cried when I hung up the phone.

And then I was mad; it was evident he had cooled on the case. We let the statute run out!

My plan for revenge—through the justice system—was crushed, and with it, my depression continued. I was mad at the attorney. I was mad at the doctors who wouldn't testify, and I was mad at everyone. Brian continued to be the one person I could trust.

Wasn't there someone, a witness—a good doctor who was willing to step forward; was there no one who could help me right this wrong!

I was denied my right to due process. As an American citizen—an American woman, I couldn't believe this!

Brian and I agree that the law in Michigan that prevents the filing of a lawsuit without attaching a physician's affidavit of merit may be an abrogation of one's right to due process, and thus unconstitutional.

In a February 25, 1999, letter to Dr. Randolph, I told him of my loss of legal redress:

When I asked my doctor why I couldn't keep my ovaries she unequivocally and unconditionally said, 'But we can put it all back' not less than three times. You have always known how untrue that statement is. I am astounded and bitterly disappointed by this unjust outcome.

My attorney contends that my legal rights have been violated—that my doctor should be held to a higher standard because of the inherent trust in a doctor/patient relationship. He is further troubled that my consent was coerced as my doctor scheduled the BSO surgery twelve days before I signed the consent form.

I know that you will be greatly relieved that this lawsuit is not going forward. I know you had no taste for it; I hated to involve you in it as you have been so good to me. However, I am a principled woman; I felt a duty to come forward!

The attorney suggested that I get on with my life, but how could I do that when I was still consumed with fury. I began to read whatever I could get my hands on about the effects of these surgeries upon women. The more I read, the more I realized that I should never have had the surgeries; I also discovered the losses I experienced were to be expected!

My doctor knew what she had done to me—how the surgery would impact my life! It is in the medical literature! Somehow I was going to get even!

In The Hysterectomy Hoax, Dr. Stanley West, a noted fertility expert, is very candid about the abuses within the profession. He says he sees doctors who either early in their residency or professional careers stop thinking of patients as people, and solicit procedures as a matter of course, even when they know they are deleterious to their patients.

In a May 4, 1999 letter to Dr. Randolph, I share that Stanley West, MD wonders how a woman can have an orgasm without a uterus. He cites Masters and Johnson. Their research showed that sexual excitement prompts the uterus to undergo a series of contractions.

"All of the other orgasms – vaginal, clitoral, and nipple are the initiators of this excitement and the contractions are the end point of the excitement and the female orgasm requires these contractions." Finally there was a full explanation of why I had lost so much of my sexual pleasure!

In a June 1, 1999 letter, I told Dr. Randolph that Dr. West states in his book, The Hysterectomy Hoax, "No woman who has had her ovaries removed will ever be the same afterwards." I was living proof. I was still grappling with the new me! Instead of life in high definition, my life was obscured.

It was like I was a bystander in my life, not a participant. There was a filter on my lens causing me to see things out of focus—abstracted, detached, diminished—shrouded in fog!

I had recent memory lapses, directional blackouts; I couldn't remember people's names; crying and depression followed me everywhere. I had lost my sense of humor, my joy in the day— my raison d'etre.

On June 20, 1999, I sent a complaint letter to the administrators at my doctor's hospital. It said:

Your hospital narrowly missed a malpractice action because as the end of the 2 year statute of limitations neared I did not have the attorney give the permitted 6 month notice of intent to sue, which would have extended the statute accordingly.

I told them of a 1992 decision in Maryland that awarded substantial damages to a woman and her husband following a TAH-BSO holding that the physician breached the standard of care by failing to warn a patient of the material risks, complications and side effects, which were inherent in the procedure, which were the proximate cause of her post surgery physical and emotional suffering, and without all of the relevant information the patient was deprived of her ability to make an informed consent about what would be done to her body.

It was a good letter; it required an answer. When I had not received a response to my letter after three months, Brian wrote to them demanding a reply to the serious allegations I had outlined. I then received a letter saying they had formed a Quality Review Committee which would look into my complaint.

A Quality Review Committee? That sounds like pure stalling.

In an August 21, 1999, letter, I told Dr. Randolph:

It is hard for me to realize that I had this surgery because I was starting to go through a normal phase of a woman's life, perimenopause. Dr. West states that as a woman approaches menopause the first hormone that the ovaries cease producing is progesterone.

He explains when this happens the periods become irregular and even women who have never had any trouble with their periods may experience mood swings, irritability and symptoms of PMS. These were the problems that brought me to my doctor in November of 1996.

It is even harder for me to realize that my request for drugs to regulate my periods was denied. I later discovered my request for a low dose birth control drug to regulate my periods was right on target and the treatment of choice by many gynecologists.

Instead hysterectomy was offered as the only solution—a permanent solution to a minor temporary problem. I know you would like to give your colleague and former student the benefit of the doubt, but I believe the facts in this case are straight forward.

I had never experienced any gynecological problems; I had never asked my doctor for help before November of 1996. I believed my doctor knew I would come to her for help at this phase of my life and it would be her opportunity to press for the surgery she had solicited and I had declined many times throughout the ten years I had gone to her.

In December of 1999, I received a response from the Quality Review Committee at my doctor's hospital. They said that they had talked to the doctor, (they didn't talk to me) and I had been informed of all of the 'risks and benefits' of the surgery and I had agreed to it. She was absolved of all wrongdoing. How can you conduct an investigation without consulting with the complainant?

The hospitals are enablers of these procedures; they want to keep their operating rooms full.

I was smoking! If there was literature clearly showing this was wrong, how could she be absolved—it was wrong, wrong, wrong.

I wanted to strike out at those who allow this injustice, but what to do and how to do it? Maybe I didn't know yet, but I wasn't going to go quietly.

8-The Secrets of the Surgeries: An Exposé

. . . .

Several weeks after the Statute of Limitations expired I was surfing the web one day and I came across the Hysterectomy Educational Resources and Services (HERS) Foundation website. I called the number and spoke with Nora Coffey, the Founder, Director and President; she spoke with me for several hours.

She asked me to send her my medical records; she knew of doctors who would be willing to be the expert witness. Could we extend the statute in Michigan? Unfortunately, that wasn't possible; we failed to file the required form that would extend the Statute for six months.

My hopes were shattered. I was crestfallen, dismayed and despondent. No one, except for Brian and now Nora, believed in me and my case enough to be my advocate. I had finally found someone who could provide an expert witness for me but I had let the attorney talk me into not filing the form that would extend the statute for six months.

We would have found the witness in the added extra time with Nora's help! I was mad at myself for letting my legal representative dissuade me in my quest for justice without giving it our best shot.

It became evident that my attorney had lost interest in the case; he let it sit; he let the statute expire. I should have insisted that he extend the statute. He should have encouraged me to find someone else to represent me while there was still time. He let me down. I let myself down.

It was hard for me to understand and accept what was done to me and why—and that there was no legal recourse. It helped to write to Dr. Randolph about it. I bared my soul to him; he didn't take it lightly. Dr. Randolph told me he did read my letters. It was a way for me to heal.

I am still steaming about my lack of due process one year later. In a letter dated February 10, 2000, I told Dr. Randolph: The medical profession believed when a woman's reproductive life was over her uterus and her ovaries were no longer necessary and they could be removed without harm, as 'excess baggage'.

This is out of date medicine. As a group doctors have a responsibility to exert pressure through continuing education to bring about change in the standard of care.

My son Andrew recently received his board certification in Orthopedic Surgery. He must renew every ten years by taking his board exams. He mentioned that this is a rather recent requirement.

He said that they grandfathered the older Orthopedic Surgeons out of having to take this periodic exam. He said he knows of some who would not be able to pass the current requirements for Board Certification.

Brian is a 1966 graduate of the University of Michigan Law School. He is an excellent attorney who has much experience; he continues to take legal continuing education seminars to keep his practice current.

If he did not dispense correct current legal advice, he could be subject to a court action. To practice the law as it existed when he graduated from law school, or even 20, 10 or 2 years ago, would not be a defense.

The same should be expected for doctors caring for female patients with so much at stake.

The quality of my life will never be the same because of a doctor who practices out of date, self serving and harmful medicine. I am outraged that my efforts for retribution within the legal system and to bring about change within the medical profession have thus far been unsuccessful.

I am furious that these self imposed impediments by the medical profession, and by legislation added at the behest of the medical profession and their insurers, through their lobbies, that deprive a woman of her right to due process, also debase her by legalizing a standard of medicine that is known to be bad medicine.

Brian told me the letter of February 10, to Dr. Randolph was too angry; he said I owed him an apology. I said, "I'll tell him when I see him next." Brian said, "That's not good enough! You need to apologize in a note." In a February 20, 2000, letter, I told Dr. Randolph:

The drugs that you have given me have not restored my sexual response to any substantial degree. I realize you can't put my organs back that were essential to my orgasmic experience.

No woman who enjoys sex would consent to these surgeries if she was truthfully told that the removal of her uterus and cervix and the shortening of her vagina would compromise her orgasmic ability.

I closed the letter with these exact words, "It is three years this May 14, since my first appointment with you. I've come a long way thanks to your help. I am fortunate to be your patient and I hope you understand my comments in my letter of February 10, and accept my apology if I offended you."

In the fall of 2000, Nora Coffey asked me to be a panelist at the HERS Twentieth Hysterectomy Conference in Philadelphia. Brian accompanied me to the Conference. Here was my opportunity to bring awareness to others of the concealed 'secrets' of these surgeries.

In an October 26, 2000 letter to Dr. Randolph, I convey to him some of what transpired during my presentation: "I tried to add a little levity to my talk and got a chuckle from the audience. I mentioned, I don't know what I was doing, a woman who raised sheep and had a llama castrated to elicit more docile behavior, to consent to the BSO."

There is nothing funny about what happened to me, but I must have been getting some of my sense of humor back at this point in time, because I could see the audience's shoulders shifting up and down; I could hear their laughter after that comment.

I shared with them that when Brian came home each night for a year after my surgery he held me on his lap while I cried. I divulged what his comments were one night, several months into this behavior, when he said, "She ruined you.", which were the last three words of my presentation; I finished with tears in my eyes.

Women came up to me afterwards and thanked me for sharing my story with them.

It helped me immeasurably to give my anger a positive spin by speaking to others. If I save just one woman from this barbaric procedure, it will be worthwhile. Speaking to women at risk gave me a sense of purpose, which in turn provided a modicum of closure for this misdeed! It was the beginning of a new chapter in my life.

I was doing better three and one half years after the surgery, but I was still teetering on a tight rope of emotional equilibrium. I still danced with my demons—each and every day. They were with me all of the time; they dwelt in me and remained because the criminal act done to me had had no retribution; they were nimble and sly, ever trying to be in the forefront.

It was a balancing act; I sequestered them in an inner room during the day, so I could push one foot in front of the other—unencumbered; they knew they were only free to surface in the darkness of my night solitude, where they subsisted on my suppressed rage.

Back in December of 1998, Dr. Randolph had put me on a .25 mg. dose of micronized methyl testosterone which, over a period of time, he gradually increased to a dosage of .75 mg. I finally stopped crying and felt better on the higher dose of testosterone, but it came with a price, adult acne and nightmares.

In my nightmares I am trying to stop my hysterectomy; I try to stop it before they remove all of my organs; especially my ovaries, I try to get up, but I am already restrained on the operating table; I am groggy; I can see the blood running from the cuts on my body. The surgery has already started! It is too late to stop them. I awaken to the real nightmare—what I now live with everyday!

Every nightmare makes me relive the terrifying moment of no return.

Brian and I believe that what was done to me was a battery on my person. We believe my physician's actions reached the level of Mens Rea, a legal term which means to have a guilty mind, a guilty or wrongful purpose; a criminal intent-- guilty knowledge and willfulness.

It was an egregious breach of trust by a fiduciary! There is lifelong resultant debilitation! There was no atonement! How does one move on?

Could I put enough of it in my past, or at least control it enough to help others.

The nightmares continually fought against anything positive.

9-In My Heart of Hearts

. . . .

One of the many good things that came of my speaking at the HERS Conference was that I began painting again. Before the surgery, there wasn't a time when I couldn't remember painting.

Creating beautiful and colorful images on paper sustained my soul. It was part of me; I needed to paint to be who I was. But I couldn't offer that part of me anymore; my emotional numbing since my surgery had left a vacuum in my font of original artistic expression.

I had a gift, a talent, which I think I inherited from my Great Uncle Joe Kraemer, who for many years was the head artist at the Detroit News, when drawing was an important part of illustrating a newspaper. He had an eye for detail. It was uncanny. It was as if Great Uncle Joe's drawings and mine were done by the same hand.

On the flight back from the HERS Conference I became acquainted with two watercolor teachers, Nita Engle and Chris Unwin, who were returning from a workshop they conducted in Philadelphia. I mentioned to Chris, "Watercolor is my passion, but I have not been able to pick up my paints." She remarked, "Come to my class tomorrow." I did.

I made myself go! I was worried that I still could not offer the part of me which saw the beauty in simple shapes and colors; I questioned if I retained, somewhere in my shattered mind and body, the unique ability to dynamically compose and complete an art work of merit! I wondered if I would fall short of whom I used to be. If I was ever going to get the old me back, I knew I had to try to paint again!

I went to Chris's class; I could see that I was out of practice; it would be a long way back to regain my former status. But coming back from this surgery, this life altering surgery—was sort of like a near death experience. I bargained for my future; I would value the time and abilities that I had left. I made a commitment to myself; I would devote a given amount of time to a former passion which I hoped would return—the love of watercolor painting!

In time I discovered that painting was therapy. It offered a place I could go, like a time capsule, where I could escape from the trauma I lived with each day. It was a venue where I found a talent, which was still there, so I fostered it, fueled it, and it nourished me.

Four years after my surgery, I was still consumed with rage over what was done to me and why. Intuitively, I realized I must channel my fury or it would destroy me.

In a letter of August 14, 2001, I told Dr. Randolph:

I am trying to direct my anger in a positive direction with my involvement with the HERS Foundation; by counseling women at risk of the surgery of the usually undisclosed negative consequences; by bringing knowledge of this damage to the medical establishment and by writing to you.

But even these positive steps don't defray my anger. Some say that anger and depression are related. I know that I will suffer from this anger/ depression for the rest of my life, not only because of my losses, but because I have a biochemical imbalance caused by the surgery.

Brian says it is difficult to live with someone who is now so angry who used to be always laughing. I am very different post-operative, which my friends confirm.

It is in the medical literature that depression follows BSO. Dr. West states in his book, The Hysterectomy Hoax, "They don't understand the depression that follows a BSO. And it does not respond to hormone therapy."

In a September 28, 2001, letter, I wrote some strong words to Dr. Randolph:

No other profession has the latitude of the medical profession. If the specialty does not take more responsibility and police their colleagues, then that privilege is undeserved.

If the surgery wasn't so radical, the injuries so acute, the damage so life altering and irreversible, one might agree it is OK to turn the other cheek. But that is not the case.

I find it very believable that you learned on your sabbatical that there is no testing on the effects of testosterone use. Prior to this surgery, I was one of the lucky ones. Sex with Brian was always a ten and even getting better with more time and opportunity now that our young fledglings are on their own.

Understandably I am angry that what was always a ten on a ten-point scale went to a two or a three, at best, post-operative. I believe with certainty that this loss of intensity of orgasm with coitus is substantially attributable to my altered anatomy and not from the loss of testosterone.

In late fall, 2001, I was back to working on our farm. The Michigan Christmas Tree Association asked if we would host a workshop that fall. I said, "Yes", knowing that it would force me to get our barn ready for Christmas.

There were two concrete stave silos at each end of the old dairy barn that needed to go. They were fifteen feet across and forty and fifty feet tall. Each was constructed of concrete staves, tongue and groove, twelve inches wide by thirty inches long, off setting, with metal rods around the outside holding them together.

I contacted a good friend, Charlie Braun, who had a license to use explosives. He agreed to do it, but said, "My hands are shaky; I have gait problems; if you want me to do it, you and Roy have to place the cartridges in the silos."

Roy and I hurriedly placed the Kenapack (dynamite and nitroglycerin) packages on the inside of the silo at the base; we joined Charlie in time as he readied the detonator.

He set off the explosion; it blew about half of the bottom staves out from under the silo. Charlie explained to us, "I need you and Roy to repeat the process." As Roy and I reentered the now undermined, but still standing silo, I joked with Roy, "I think I know why Charlie's hands are shaking—maybe it has nothing to do with his gait problem?"

This time the explosion took out all but one of the cement concrete blocks. The silo was standing on one stave. Charlie said, "We needed one more package of explosives." I shrieked, "We can't go back in there!" As we were debating our next plan of action, the silo imploded to the ground in a roar. We took down the other silo on our first attempt!

On that bright sunny afternoon, there were lessons learned. ... I hadn't fully assessed the danger. ... Did I endanger Roy?

As for my life in danger, there had been, in my heart of hearts, a loss of verve for life since my surgery. It was not an intellectual loss, but a physical/emotional--gut reaction loss, the visceral feeling of being there—on the edge—involved in life to the fullest.

I had finally gotten over the thoughts of suicide but there were times when I didn't care about danger! I had never been a risk taker. Since the surgery, I didn't care about a safety net.

It wasn't so much that I was reckless, it was more of the realization that I didn't have to worry about the worst thing that could ever happen to me in life, because it already had!

So it was interesting to me that I balked at reentering the silo. With the possibility of facing a violent death, I chose life!

In the fall of 2001, I was invited back to speak at the HERS Foundation's Twenty-First Conference in Philadelphia. The Keynote Speaker, Dr. Lopa A. Meta, an Indian physician, spoke on: Violence in Medicine; Gynecology's Role in Causing Damage and Disease in Women.

Prior to my surgery, I was timid about flying—I would rather take the train! But I got on a plane several weeks after 9/11; I would take my chances; I needed to spread the word. I prepared and did a better job of speaking! Brian told me, "You were great!"

I couldn't have done any of this without Brian's help. My sense of direction was slow to return. He accompanied me to the conferences. In the beginning he was one of the few men in attendance. I needed his support and love to spread my wings again—he offered it mightily.

After speaking at the conference, a feeling of calmness and closure settled in me. I knew that my talk was compelling—convincing! I knew women were saved that day from a surgery that may have harmed them as it did me. I had made the difference. I was empowered!

As I came away from this second conference, where I had spoken so well, I knew that I had made another commitment to myself that day. I would continue to reach out to women in this way.

Speaking to women was my healing—that and writing to Dr. Randolph; these were both ways that I could make a difference; I wanted to reach him as an educator in hopes that significant change might come about in teaching about this practice— this practice of maiming of women for profit!

10-Violence in Medicine

. . . .

Victims of violence are often trusting of the person who commits the crime.

Keynote Speaker Dr. Lopa A. Meta's presentation at the 21st HERS Conference was about violence in medicine, specifically gynecologist's role in aiding and abetting it. She explained, "In India, there is much less gynecological intervention; and statistically women do just as well, maybe better."

Those were strong words! I thought about the validity of her comments and how they particularly pertained to my own personal experience. It had taken all of this time for me to realize the scope of all of my new limitations, disabilities and losses, and to fully comprehend that I was victimized.

After listening to other victims of this violence, I began to see similarities in what they experienced after the crime, and my reaction to discovering deliberate unnecessary surgery. We share a loss of status, a sense of betrayal, rage, the inability to move past the transgression, and we are unable to forgive the perpetrator. I am convinced I am suffering from Post Traumatic Stress Disorder (PTSD); I wonder if it may be the cause of my nightmares.

Be it a date rape, or a pedophile priest sexually abusing a child, the victims often are trusting of the person who commits the crime, making it even more difficult for the victim to sort out the reasons for the assault and betrayal.

I can't help but see the parallels. I consider what happened to me to be analogous to the pedophile priest scandal in the Catholic Church. I see little difference between the harm done to the young victims of sexual abuse and women who are exploited by having had essential body parts unnecessarily removed—for profit.

Like the young molested children, women—gynecologists' victims--can only begin the healing when this practice is exposed for what it is and the violators are contrite, apologize and step down.

I cry out in the night from my nightmares. I am suffering still. These are horrible things that gynecologists do to women. Can you imagine removing a man's testicles, shortening his penis, removing nerve endings and a major blood supply to his genital area, and expecting him to function sexually again, to feel that he is a man, even with supplemental male hormones!

Yet gynecologists do this to women every day and send them home to sort it all out; to live the rest of their lives without experiencing orgasm, emotionally, physically and intellectually bankrupt.

What makes this realization, the nightmares, the losses, so incredulous to me is to see my former gynecologist resume this practice, unscathed. There was no justice!

Apparently the doctors at my former gynecologist's hospital still view hysterectomy as the "solution" to women's health problems. The doctors and the administrators at the hospital leant no credence to my complaint regarding the egregious treatment by my former gynecologist.

How are women ever going to get the medical profession to change a standard of care that is so permissive to the gynecologist; one that absolves atrocities and criminal acts performed upon women for profit.

In December of 2002, I had a phone interview with ABC News Medical Producer, Susan Wagner, who had gotten my name from Nora Coffey. I knew she understood the unfortunate consequences of the surgeries. She told me she was working on a segment for the ABC program 20/20 about hysterectomy, which was to air in the spring. It was to be about sexual dysfunction following the surgery.

I spoke with Susan at length about my personal experience being just that—sex was disappointing post surgery. Susan asked if Brian and I would come to New York to be interviewed by ABC Medical Correspondent, Dr. Tim Johnson, for the segment. I was elated! My voice would be heard.

Susan said my story was similar to many she had heard. She told me she had spoken with many physicians who corroborated these facts but none agreed to be interviewed.

The 20/20 interview was the morning of February 5, 2003. ABC flew us to New York the afternoon of February 4. We were waiting at the gate for our flight out of Metro to LaGuardia; it was announced there would be an hour and a half delay. As we sat waiting for the flight my excitement and anxiousness over this opportunity to be on ABC's 20/20 built.

It was late when we arrived at the Lucerne, a small boutique hotel at 79th and Amsterdam; I was beside myself about being in New York; it seemed surreal—our reasons for being there and what the next morning would bring. I forgot my tooth brush and ended up not getting one until morning. I wouldn't even use Brian's.

The next morning as we readied ourselves for the short walk to 147 Columbus Avenue to ABC News we were apprehensive. Brian put on a sport coat and tie. I slipped into a navy blazer, slacks and a silk turtle neck. We both looked professional even though we had never done anything like this before.

The interview with Dr. Tim, as he told us to call him, went very well. He interviewed us for an hour and a half. He is a professional; he put us at ease. I told him what had happened to bring me to these surgeries and the lifelong damage they afforded me. I was very candid about my sex life pre and post operative. Dr. Johnson asked good questions, for which I had good answers.

At the end of the interview Dr. Tim raised his fist, looked at the producer and said, "Now we have to fight." I assumed that meant for the story, to present it in full.

Susan came up to me afterwards; she said, "You were terrific; you did an outstanding job." She told Brian that the camera crew said, "It was an excellent interview." Susan smiled as she confided, "They are the experts."

I was pleased with Susan's comments. I had given it my best shot. I was glad that she was pleased; the camera crew told us personally that it was a really good interview. It was apparent that Dr. Tim thought so too!

Susan insisted on some footage for what they call a 'B roll'. I balked at this at first, because I felt if I was only going to have a few minutes to discuss hysterectomy/oophorectomy, and that was the reason I had come to New York, that all of the time should be spent doing that.

She said, "TV is like a magazine. We need some pictures of you and Brian." We went to a Folk Art Museum and then to Central Park for the filming. Susan and I talked all the way to Central Park. We had an instant rapport.

We laughed about my forgetting my toothbrush. She said, "You should have called

Housekeeping." Then she chuckled, "Imagine having the courage to talk about the quality of your orgasms on National TV and being too faint hearted to use your husband's toothbrush."

Brian and I took a few extra days in New York; we had a delightful time; it was a different city than we remembered from thirty plus years before. We saw an incredibly moving video about 9/11 at the New York City Historical Museum and visited many world class museums.

I was so glad I had come to New York; I could only hope my doctor would be in the National Audience—watching! I would be vindicated!

The 20/20 segment was to air in March, but the Iraq War preempted it.

I still didn't know if I had made the cut! Would we be in Susan's segment? Would I be able to reach this National Audience whom I so wanted to reach?

I would be crushed if it didn't air—it would steal my piece of vindication against my violator.

11-20/20

. . . .

What happened to me was like a date rape! I was a victim of a violent act, perpetrated by somebody I trusted. Since this unfortunate event, in order to make some sense of my life, I reached out to other women who were at risk of incurring the same violence.

It was a direction in life I would not have chosen to follow, but it was one which I now found I had no choice but to follow. Brian's life had changed course, too! Because I had not completely regained my sense of direction—my bearings—especially in new venues, he volunteered to accompany me on my missions: to bring public awareness to the pitfalls of these surgeries, the abuse of doctors' authority, and the inequities in due process.

I'm sure it was not the path he would have chosen either! But the course of our lives together had changed; our marriage was rerouted; I knew a lot of husbands who would not have stayed; he knew I needed him. He loved me; he was steadfast!

I believed Brian could see the benefit I received from my participating--spreading the word of how deleterious these surgeries are to women. He went beyond what an ordinarily good husband would do. He picked up my cause and made it his own.

He became an activist too! When the opportunity arose, he would tell how hysterectomy and / or castration affected the husband.

A fair amount of his leisure time, and travel time, where he might have preferred to be fly fishing, hunting with our son John, or at a football game, he was there for me, helping me get better, supporting in whatever way he could.

When Nora Coffey asked me to join her to give a talk to the medical students at the University of Pittsburgh Medical School in the fall of 2002, Brian drove me to Pittsburgh.

In March of 2003, Nora asked me to speak with her to several Women's Studies Classes, at the University of Pennsylvania, Westchester Campus. Brian and I flew to Philadelphia. We rented a car and drove to Nora's home in Bala Cynwyd, PA.

I was painting again. I had given my first watercolor painting to Dr. Randolph for his help. Now I carried another to Nora. I wanted to thank her for providing therapy for me--involving me in her Foundation. The painting was a field of flowers. Nora's home held many lovely paintings. She was pleased with the painting. She said, "I'll hang it with the others." I had found the perfect gift. It was healthy to be painting again; it was nice to be able to give back a little for what I had been given.

Brian and I stayed in Wayne, PA that trip. I remember that when we got to our hotel, after leaving Nora's house, we flipped on the TV to hear of the imminent invasion of Iraq, which began that night.

Wayne was a short drive from Valley Forge. We managed to work in a tour. It was so interesting and moving. Some of the very rustic troop accommodations still remain. Those that survived were obviously tough. I could relate!

In July, Susan Wagner called to say that the show was on! And we were a part of it. She wanted to come to the farm for some B roll. ABC had hired a free lance photographer crew from the Detroit area. They spent most of the day at our farm getting the pictures she wanted for the segment.

It was a day I will never forget. I couldn't believe I was going to be in the National spotlight. ABC News was coming to our farm! I was thrilled, excited, nervous and more than a little apprehensive.

I welcomed telling my story—sharing it with women. I wasn't daunted at the prospect of such a large local and National audience. My hopes to bring about change in a bad practice had a chance of coming to fruition.

The 20/20 segment aired on August 22, 2003. Brian and I saw most of our part of the segment that morning on Good Morning America, where it was shown as a promotion for that evening's 20/20 show.

There was a clip of our Christmas Tree Farm sign with the telephone number on it—on National television. The phone started to ring immediately; calls from as far away as Texas and California came from damaged women.

The flurry of calls subsided as the day continued. The stories of the women with whom I spoke were the same as my story, with some variations. We commiserated. It legitimized my reaction to what had happened to me.

Brian and I were pleased to be a part of Susan's well done show. She told us we would not be disappointed; it was everything she said it would be. I had been worried about how we would be portrayed.

I had tried to get an article about what happened to me in the local newspaper and the reporter would not let me see what she had written about my experience. The young woman was doing an internship at the paper. The story never came about. Her editor vetoed it.

I couldn't put myself and Brian in the position of being subject to ridicule. I knew we were taking a chance. But Susan told me she was a professional and she was. There was no need to have worried.

It was a courageous move on my part—to talk about my sexual experience on National TV. In a letter to Dr. Randolph I told him, "We thought Susan's segment was provocative and educational; her handling of the sensitive nature of the program seemed tastefully done."

It was worth taking the chance. Our kids called to say they were proud of us; Lynda said, "Gynecologists have to start listening to women!"

Both of my parents are gone now, but I wonder what my mother and my father would have thought of their daughter being part of a National TV Program. I know both of my parents would have been disappointed that I succumbed to a ploy, albeit in part because of their old fashioned teaching on following doctors' orders precisely, but I think they would have been proud that I moved forward in the way that I had.

I come from a line of strong women. My mother was a fighter; she took advantage of every opportunity offered; she got an education; she fought her way out of a one horse town; she bucked the odds and rose above her humble beginnings.

My mother always taught me to respect myself and my body. She taught me it was not always the easy way, but the correct way. I'm sure that is why I followed the course that I followed with my doctor after the surgery.

When you are a young woman, I don't think you want to be like your mother, to emulate her. I know I didn't. I found my mother imposing. I have come to realize that I am my mother—a fighter—a woman with an agenda, to right a wrong!

Some of our friends and even people whom we didn't know that well, who watched the 20/20 segment, said I came across as a strong and angry woman. I knew that I must comment on this disrespectful practice and treatment of women and I was grateful for having had the opportunity.

I find that I am now the Matriarch of our fine family. I feel a responsibility to carry on its tradition.

12-Uniformed Consent

. . . .

I know they know they are wrong—doctors who perform these surgeries—they know they do harm to women—they hear it from woman after woman!

I brought Dr. Randolph a copy of U of M Bio-Ethicist Carl Schneider's book, The Practice of Autonomy; Patients, Doctors, and Medical Decisions; I asked him, "How can doctors who take the Hippocratic Oath, to above all do no harm, routinely remove healthy, essential body parts from women? How could my doctor who got caught doing what she did to me come through it unscathed?"

He shared with me that my former doctor's practice is 'temperate' because of my case. It certainly was no consolation compared with the torture I had been put through.

Nora Coffey planned a protest of hysterectomy in every state in the Union, from March of 2004, through March of 2005 culminating with a protest in Washington, D.C. In a September 8, 2004 letter to Dr. Randolph, I told him about the Detroit protest, which was at St. Joseph Mercy Hospital in Pontiac.

I told him I found it difficult to protest; it was something I had never done. Before this surgery I was a private person. I wasn't comfortable attracting attention. Brian was more at ease approaching people. He was a wonderful protestor.

A senior hospital administrator came out and asked him, "Why our hospital? We are a Catholic hospital. We don't do unnecessary hysterectomies." He told her, "You have a sister hospital in Ann Arbor; they routinely perform unnecessary hysterectomies."

One female protestor who had gone through the same ordeal was approached by a male gynecologist who said he did not do unnecessary hysterectomies and would report anyone at their hospital who did.

He asked if she filed a grievance with the State about her case. She told him that both she and I filed a grievance with the State Licensing Board and that neither doctor was rebuked. He hurried on his way without further ado.

The protesting women talked about informed consent. HERS Foundation has pertinent data that 99.7% of the 800,000 women it has counseled since it's inception in 1982 report that they had not received the information necessary to give an informed consent prior to their surgery.

The protest was empowering. I will never look at protestors in quite the same way. The Detroit protest was the day of our 40th wedding anniversary. Brian was walking the streets with me in the rain. I needed his support in this terrible journey that gave me self-doubt. He assumed whatever role he needed to be there for me. He never let me down.

Dr. Randolph and I talked at our appointment on September 29, 2004. In a follow up letter of the next day I wrote:

I have to rebut what you had to say about the 8 billion dollar a year business of hysterectomy. It is not OK to allow attrition to curb this abuse of women.

You mentioned that what I am doing and you are doing by educating women is the best way to reform. But we reach so few women; we are up against big business; and the complexities and trust inherent in an often long-term doctor patient relationship.

You postulated that because it is within the standard of care to perform these surgeries to treat non-life threatening health issues of women, therefore there isn't much that can be done to initiate change.

Standard of care is the threshold of acceptable medicine; it is the minimum level of care required to avoid exposure to a claim of malpractice. Doctors write the Standard of Care. I suggested to Dr. Randolph, "We need good doctors to rewrite it."

He mentioned that insurers hope to curtail unnecessary hysterectomies by requiring second opinions, but often the second opinion is to proceed with the surgery. I said, "That's why we need legal restrictions on them."

I had good insurance. I wrote to Blue Cross Blue Shield telling them what had happened to me. I got a form letter back. It seems they are glad to remove every thing they can—they think it prevents future problems, but they don't connect the trail of doctors a woman then frequents after the surgery to the surgery.

Dr. Randolph also cautioned me that there are no long term studies on testosterone use; his goal is to minimize the drugs I take in the future with the long range plan to eliminate them entirely.

I realize the unknown dangers posed by the drugs I am taking; the surgery essentially took the decision away from me; I find I am forced to take them. I am livid that an unnecessary surgery has placed me in such a jeopardized position—I was not presented with these facts by my former gynecologist. I would never have consented to be subject to drugs that pose potential health risks.

The decision to take these drugs is a quality of life decision. It is my decision; I will weigh it carefully. I know that if I go back to where I was for many years after my surgery, I won't care how long I live, but I now know there is a caveat.

In October 2004, I watched a broadcast of David Suzuki's CBC The Nature of Things, Sex Lies and Secrecy; Dissecting Hysterectomy. It gave some troubling statistics. Three quarters of a million hysterectomies are performed in North America each year, five times the rate of Europe, where it appears health care for women is more conservative! Essentially, there is less of the fee for service medicine in Europe.

The bottom line is the surgery is cruel–a castration of women, and as I've mentioned before, would men want this surgery if they were getting castrated?

In the early 1800s, the practice of castrating the Castrati Singers was discontinued due to the severe health and emotional problems which resulted.

And yet in 2004, 78% of women are castrated at the time of surgery, with less than 2% of the surgeries performed for cancer. With suspected cancer, organ sparing surgery should be the norm, like the use of lumpectomy for breast cancer, in lieu of radical mastectomy.

Psychiatrist Dr. Lorraine Dennerstien, at the University of Melbourne, who holds a PhD in hormones and behavior, explained that when the cervix is removed the nerves that run up the spine to the brain are severed resulting in a loss of feeling in the clitoris, labia, vagina and nipples.

Lise Cloutier-Steele, author of an anthology of seventeen courageous women entitled, Misinformed Consent felt 'bullied by her surgeon'; she found The pathology report indicated her removed organs were normal; that HRT was ineffective for her, plus had many side effects of which she was not forewarned—just like me.

April 15, 2005, was the Twenty-Fourth HERS Conference and Protest in Washington D.C. The women came from all over the United States; despite their diversity in their ethnicity, socio economic status, age and education levels, the outcome of the surgeries for all was very similar.

I found some of the salient commonalities striking. Many women attendees who had had the surgery remembered the exact time, day, month and year of their surgery no matter how much time had elapsed. It is marked by all as another birthday, not a celebratory one, but the beginning date of a new and radically changed life.

An inordinate amount of these women, who had been in the arts, discovered after the surgery that their ability to perform was compromised. They were not able to participate creatively. For many it was possible to resume some of these artistic activities after many years, perhaps with therapy, but for others the passion or ability never returned.

It was four years after my surgery before I could pick up my paints again. I have changed; I bring different things to the painting, but I am now able to paint; I have a passion for it again.

I believe it is because of Dr. Randolph's kindness and care that I have come back to this degree. I am one of the luckier ones. At the Conference when keynote speaker, Barbara Seaman, asked for a poll of the attendees who felt abused by their treatment from a doctor, a majority of hands went up, including mine.

When she asked how many in the audience felt they had received extraordinary treatment from a physician post operative, a sprinkling of hands went up, mine among them. In a majority of those cases, it was not from their original doctor.

The letters I have written to Dr. Randolph have been therapeutic for me. It helps enormously to put to written words what happened to me. It makes it tangible—to see the words in print. I'm thankful to Dr. Randolph. Somehow it is healing and I knew it intuitively; I started putting my thoughts down on paper almost immediately after my surgery.

On August 1, 2005, my friend Sheila sent me a New York Times article by Richard A. Friedman, MD., entitled, I'm Sorry, which I shared with Dr. Randolph, "Many Lawyers would disagree, but doctors ought to let their patients know when they've erred, it humanizes them and builds trust."

Sheila believed an apology from my doctor early on in my case could have diffused the entire thing. I initially told Dr. Randolph I thought it would have helped.

Brian disagreed, "I lived with you through the aftermath of your surgery and I acutely remember your anger and sense of betrayal by your former gynecologist soon after your surgery."

I thought about it all day. In a follow up letter of the same day, I told Dr. Randolph that I couldn't forgive my doctor with an 'I'm sorry', "The crux of the issue is that I did not give an informed consent—nothing I experienced was as she described it would be."

I don't believe I would have accepted an apology from her had it been given; this was not a mistake, but a deliberate and malicious act. It might have been nice to hear her say 'I'm Sorry', but an apology could never diffuse my justifiable rage.

As Dr. Friedman concludes, "In the end, most patients will forgive their doctor for an error of the head, but rarely for one of the heart."

I shared another New York Times article on informed consent with Dr. Randolph in a January 31, 2006, letter:

Dr. Alan Tait, of the University of Michigan, Department of Anesthesiology, is working with colleagues to develop a simpler form. Using friendlier language is just the first step.

While simpler forms are worthwhile, nothing could ever replace the bond of trust between a doctor and a patient that is crucial to good care and is forged only during the give and take of a good conversation.

I found the conversation did not work for me; it didn't happen. There was a conversation, a more than biased one. She scheduled the surgery before I even agreed to it. My doctor grossly misrepresented the surgery; she interfered with and prevented my being adequately informed before my surgery in 1997.

During the conversation I was repeatedly told my life would be forever improved. Instead the quality of my life is forever marred. I wonder if I will ever again be able to face the day with the same semblance of whom I used to be.

Not only was my consent an uninformed consent, it was a misinformed consent.

It is so unfair; my doctor came through this breach of trust, this criminal act of violence, this misdeed, unscathed. It is doubtful that I will come through this ordeal with the same outcome.

The magnitude of what was done to me; the inequity of the outcome of my quest for closure, is something with which I still do battle; I seek an answer—justice—with such ferocity that it is hard for me to proceed yet, each and every day! It is a millstone around my neck.

I carry my burden, not lightly, but with deliberation throughout my waking hours; it is a scourge; it anchors my soul each day—it keeps my spirit leashed—it no longer soars, as it once did!

It is during the dreaded night where my struggle with my loss, my grief and my outrage is all consuming to me. It is center stage. I can barely carry the weight of it during the hours before the dawn—the anger, the injustice—what was done to me; constant reminders of my maiming are ever present.

It retreats slowly, ever so slowly, with the dawn. And I rise to greet the new day, impinged and fettered.

13-The Double Standard

. . . .

By my generation, a woman's interest and enjoyment in sex was expected—both partners were to share in the enjoyment—they would both be orgasmic! Women's sexuality was not only openly acknowledged, but affirmed!

There was the advent of safe and effective birth control (the pill); and women were becoming more enlightened.

As a young wife in 1964, I read Masters and Johnson's, Human Sexual Response. In the 1970s, I read the National Bestseller, The Joy of Sex; A

Gourmet Guide to Love Making, which I shared with Brian. Sex was an important part of our life.

The women's movement demanded more equality in the work force; women also made strides on other fronts; our personal and sexual lives were to be equal, too! So it was surprising to me that I was not told that this surgery would impair my sexual response! It just didn't happen!

There was a duty to impart this information. It is in the medical literature that more than one third of the women questioned about their sexual response post operative report a loss of status of sexual enjoyment.

It was a woman who withheld this information from me—kept this secret of the surgery!

With sex being such an important part of our lives, any woman's life, it was completely wrong she didn't inform me.

In a May 26, 2000, letter, I told Dr. Randolph: "I firmly believe the failure of the Medical Profession to advise a woman of the potential loss of sexual enjoyment with these surgeries further exemplifies the Medical Profession's male dominated teaching and dreadfully needs to be updated, which I believe you agreed to at our appointment."

The irony of this situation is that doctors weigh at great length the decision to remove a man's ability to perform and enjoy his sex life. The consequences are carefully disclosed, weighed and considered when facing a life threatening illness, but they castrate and hysterectomize his wife without a corresponding disclosure, thus compromising his sex life as well. A responding partner is a necessary ingredient to sexual enjoyment in a mutually satisfying and loving relationship.

In 2005, five years later, there still lingers some stereotypical inference—maybe women's organs and their sexual experience are of lesser importance and harder to understand than men's!

In an August 18, 2005, letter I shared with Dr. Randolph an article about the FDA's reluctance to allow marketing of the testosterone patch for women, which exemplified ample ignorance regarding a woman's sexual know-how! The article stated:

"Women's sexuality is complex, affected more deeply than men's sex drive by mood, self esteem and relationship issues. It took years for the FDA and experts to devise ways to measure improvements in a woman's libido and many still argue that counting 'satisfying sexual events' is a gauge better suited to men than to women."

How outrageous! ... Both men and women have the capacity for orgasm based upon the same physiologic responses!

Nora Coffey invited Brian to New York the last weekend in February, 2006, to meet with her, her associate Rick Schweickert, prominent New York attorney Sybil Shainwald and attorney and bio-ethicist John Merz, of the University of Penn Medical School. This time I was the tag along spouse.

The purpose of the meeting was to brainstorm about how to improve the process of informed consent. After tossing about many ideas as to how to improve the process, Rick and Nora came up with the idea of an interactive video, with viewing as a mandatory prerequisite to the consent process.

We all left the meeting sure that we had come up with the solution—but how to implement it was the next hurdle!

While in New York, Brian and I took the opportunity to meet Susan Wagner, the ABC Producer, for an extended lunch. She commented, "I chose you because you were a safe call! The climate has changed so much at ABC since we did that special, I don't think I could get approval for it today." My guess is her 20/20 segment may have been controversial; it may have not been well received by those who perform these surgeries.

My daughter-in-law, Deb, who has friends who go to my former doctor, told me her practice was not tempered by my case; she is still promoting these surgeries. I told this to Dr. Randolph. His response was, "There is so much money at stake!"

I was surprised and saddened with his comment. Money is not an excuse to allow a doctor who is known to have misused a woman, to continue a practice which abuses other woman.

I had been speaking at the HERS Conferences every fall since my first conference in 2000. The women presenters agreed; their doctors painted a rosy picture to them. I quote one who said, "The way my doctor described the surgery, it sounded as benign as having my teeth whitened."

At the Twenty-Fifth Conference in Nashville, TN, on October 28, 2006, I spoke on a panel with two much younger women. The first woman to speak was only twenty nine at the time of her TAH-BSO surgery.

Her male gynecologist started recommending the surgery to her for endometriosis, when she was only twenty five years old. She got pregnant and had a child; he then promoted the surgery again, but she was soon pregnant with her second child.

After the birth of her third child, he did exploratory surgery, which he said confirmed his claims of severe endometriosis. He performed a TAH-BSO; it was bogus. There was no endometriosis.

She said the loss of her uterine orgasms was huge. She sued and won—but her life was irreparably damaged! She finished her talk with the query, "I just want to know why! Why did he do it?" It is a question all women ask after they've been violated

At the end of the conference, a man got up to speak. He said, "From the stories I have heard today, I wonder if the gynecologists of the women who spoke are sociopaths?"

After the conference, I asked Brian, "Now do you understand what happened to me?" He answered, "I understood a long time ago! It is barbaric!"

Like the first woman who spoke at the conference, I just want to know why too; "Why did she do this to me?" It was a question I asked Brian every day I was suffering during those first few years after my surgery: It is a question I ask myself yet, everyday!

14-Knowledge Is Power

. . . .

I have always known how important grandmothers are, but not so much as I've discovered recently. One of the wonderful things that happened to me over the last ten years is that I became Nana to five wonderful little people who have magically entered their way into my heart.

There are grandsons Max, Jack, Nick and Will, in descending order of age. And the last one, finally, a granddaughter, Ali; they are all like the children in Garrison Keillor's (of a Prairie Home

Companion fame) Lake Wobegon; they are all above average.

I am sorry that they didn't have the opportunity to know me before my surgery; they will never have the full measure of their grandmother, and it stirs a pain in me to know I can't give them what I would have been able to without the surgery!

March 4, 2009, was the observance of my twelfth anniversary—an anniversary not celebrated like a birthday, but it was a birthday, marked by sadness—of when this interloper, this stranger, this visitor took up residence in my body!

When I picked up my medical records In July of 1997, I read the doctor's account of my six-week postoperative appointment, "She feels that there is a shield between her and the world. Is really quite angry that she even went ahead with the surgery. Particularly upset that she consented to have her ovaries removed. Feels as though she has been maimed."

I was maimed! I knew it immediately! I was emotionally, intellectually, and physically bereft! I hadn't been given permission to have sex yet—not until after the six week check up, so I was yet to understand that I was also sexually maimed. It was, as Brian said, barbarism!

I was sorry immediately after the surgery that I had removed my organs—so intimately connected to the core of my being! Dr. Randolph told me I hadn't come to terms with the surgery. I hadn't! I was pressured, hurried, bullied—coerced!

When I called my doctor seven weeks after my surgery to complain that nothing was as she described it would be, I confronted her about my sex life. I told her that the surgery had ruined it. She said, sarcastically, "It gets better."

That is a lie! When the nerves were cut that connected my organs at the cervix to my brain, I experienced exactly what Dr. Dennerstien explained on the CBC broadcast, The Nature of Things. There was a loss of feeling in my clitoris, labia, vagina and nipples.

But the most demonstrative and devastating loss to me was the loss of my uterine orgasm. I understand that less than half of all women experience uterine orgasms. So for those who do not experience the contractions of the uterus at orgasm, the loss of the uterus may not be that significant.

But for women who did experience these contractions of the uterus at orgasm, like me—this total body experience, which was felt from the top of my head to the tip of my toes, and which

I considered my ultimate end point to the sexual excitement; failing to have this experience after my surgery was a devastating loss, as I'm sure it is to all women who had it.

The doctors don't listen; they even mock and laugh, but they know! Each night, in the wee hours after I fall asleep, the nightmare unfolds. I review the course of events which brought me to whom I am today—this visitor--so much less than I was.

It is as fresh as if it had happened that day. I resurrect the images of the surgery, the losses, the betrayal, the anger and the angst. I try to get the images to recede, but they are ever there—in my inner turmoil.

I still awake in anguish crying out why? Why did I allow someone to ruin me?

I know this ritual will not end for me while I have a breath left in my body. I will never get over what another human being—a woman—did to me for profit, or empowerment, or just because she could—it is allowed!

If you look at an X-ray of a woman who has been castrated and hysterectomized, you will see the ganglia of severed nerves, hanging limply in the empty cavity where her organs once resided.

They had connected to her removed organs; they ran their course up her spine to her brain, where they affected every cell in her body. My physician son tells me when you sever connections to the brain you impact the function of the brain; it is forever different! So there is the explanation! There you have it, and it is horrible!

The last twelve years have proven a love story! Brian has been there for me. He stayed; our marriage survived! He did mean it when he said for better or for worse.

It is as if what we have been through together the last twelve years has strengthened our love, our marriage. It required not only commitment from Brian, but sacrifice—not just for the short term, but every day since.

I realize what he did for me. I know he is a special husband. The bond between us is more than many couples have. Our love was tested! We came through adversity! We endured an ordeal together; we triumphed!

I am grateful for our life together, our lovely family, our good friends; I am lucky that I was able to recharge my passion for watercolor painting; my work on the farm was met with success and I've escaped the wicked grasp of depression and I am once again glad for my life!

I am grateful to Dr. Randolph, the recipient of so many of my letters. Early in our doctor/patient relationship, I told him in a letter of August 21, 1999, that I believed fate played a role in our lives. "It was my karma. I also believe it was your fate to have me for a patient."

Dr. Randolph is a generous and compassionate physician. I believe he read my letters! He is an intelligent man and a receptive doctor. I know he learned from me, and I learned from him, too.

Another one who helped me greatly over the last twelve years was Nora Coffey. It was therapeutic for me to be involved in her Foundation, and to be fortunate enough to have Susan Wagner choose me as a participant for her well done 20/20 segment was empowering to me when I needed it—not everyone is so lucky. I got to my audience!

You know some of the woman I was before the surgery—I'm back to an extent. My grit is what kept me going in those dark days after the surgery when I could barely function. It never really left me! It buoyed me!

I endured indignity; I was humbled; I experienced gender discrimination for the first time in my life—I was a victim of malpractice, but I was denied my day in court—I believed I was denied justice because I was a woman; my body parts did not have enough societal value for a physician to sign an affidavit of merit. I wonder what testicles are worth?

I knew how wrong this was; I was betrayed by someone who held my trust—a fiduciary who owed me a duty to provide good care—someone who had taken an oath, "Above all do no harm".

It was my dogged determination, my tenacity, my anger and my resolve which caused me to devolve into the person I am today; it causes me to chip away at these acts of violence and crimes against women. I have fought my way to try to bring public awareness to the magnitude of this wrongdoing.

I accept any opportunity which I have to educate women. Brian and I accompanied Nora Coffey and her associate, Rick Schweikert, to a Women and Gender Conference at the University of Connecticut, in February of 2007. We all (Hysterectomy affects the husband, too!) spoke at a round table discussion.

We had another opportunity to speak in June of 2007, in St. Charles, Ill, at the National Women's Studies Association Conference, where we again were able to reach young women, and several women's educators, too.

We have to start with programs in the schools. Young women should be taught to revere their bodies; they should be taught their organs are not expendable.

I want my granddaughter, Ali, to have safe alternatives for the common gynecological problems that now routinely take our germane, female, sexual organs. I want her to spend her life as an intact human being so she may avail herself to all that life has to offer.

Women need to be strong; they need to fight for their rights; they need to understand the role of these organs. These sex organs are integral to women; they are lifelong guardians of women. Women need to embrace their gender!

Stanley West, M D, told Dr. Tim Johnson on the 20/20 Hysterectomy Sexual Dysfunction segment, when asked, "How are we going to stop this 'just take it out' mentality?" He answered, "Women! Women are the ones who will change this practice!"

He is right. Women will be the ones. I am one of them.

Knowledge is Power!

Afterword

. . . .

Andrew told me that physicians who obtain a patient's signature on a consent form may falsely believe they have satisfied all requirements of an informed consent.

That is not the case if the patient has not been given all of the relevant information necessary to be fully apprised of what will be done to their body and of the possible and probable effects of same.

A doctor breaches the standard of care by failing to worn a patient of all of the material risks, side effects and complications which are inherent in a procedure.

Depression is inherent in a TAH-BSO surgery. A loss of sexual status is inherent in a TAH-BSO surgery. I was not advised of either of these by my doctor. She had a duty to do so.

Even if I had been told more of what I was going to experience with these surgeries, I could not have been able to comprehend the suffering and loss. The loss of sexual feeling is huge.

Depression is incomprehensible to anyone who has not experienced it, and up until my surgery I had not.

It has been twelve years since I first encountered its clutching, choking grip. I was robbed of my essence—my inner self, my life as I had known it, my raison d'etre.

I embarked on a voyage of self destruction. I was hollowed—no longer a whole intact human being. I slumped to a place I had never been. I was a stranger to myself, a bystander.

But somewhere in my splintered mind and body I found the ability to stretch—the strength and fortitude to reach out and overcome the worst that can happen—a loss of self worth.

My rage over what was done to me will never subside. It festers and languishes in my tattered soul. It spews forth rawness. It envelops me; I walk a tight rope each day; and at night terror reigns.

I understand anger is related to depression—they are intertwined—one and the same.

But rage is not passive like depression. Rage can be positive! To channel my fury in part, I wrote this memoir of a defaced woman.

I hope reform in women's health care is on the horizon. As Rick Schweikert commented, in the near future these surgeries that debase women need to be a procedure in medicine of the past—like lobotomy.

Biography

. . . .

Susan Urquhart's first effort at authorship is a true story precipitated by a life altering event—which she was compelled to put down on paper.

She is a native Michiganian, a former middle school teacher, with a Masters degree in children's reading.

For the last 36 years she has owned and operated a Christmas tree farm near Ann Arbor, MI, where she lives with her husband, Brian, her small flock of sheep and her llama, Willie.

She has two grown sons, Andrew and John, four grandsons and a granddaughter who do "come over the river and through the woods to grandmother's house we go."